SEXUAL WELLBEING

Self-Development

Relaxation &

Rejuvenation

BY

DR. SCOTT MIKE

CONTENTS

• **INTRODUCTION**

As per the ebb and flow working definition, sexual wellbeing is a condition of physical, close to home, mental and social prosperity comparable to sexuality; it isn't only the shortfall of infection, brokenness or sickness. Sexual wellbeing requires a positive and deferential way to deal with sexuality and sexual connections, as well as the chance of having pleasurable and safe sexual encounters, liberated from pressure, separation and savagery. For sexual wellbeing to be achieved and kept up with, the sexual freedoms, everything being equal, should be regarded, safeguarded and satisfied.

Sexuality

Sexual wellbeing can't be characterized, comprehended or made functional without a wide thought of sexuality, which underlies significant ways of behaving and results connected with sexual wellbeing. The functioning meaning of sexuality is a focal part of being human over the course of life envelops sex, orientation characters and jobs, sexual direction, sensuality, delight, closeness and generation. Sexuality is capable and offered in viewpoints, dreams, wants, convictions, mentalities, values, ways of behaving, practices, jobs and connections. While sexuality can incorporate these aspects, not every one of them are constantly capable or communicated. Sexuality is affected by the association of organic, mental, social, financial, political, social, lawful, verifiable, strict and profound elements.

Sexual privileges

There is a developing agreement that sexual wellbeing can't be accomplished and kept up with without regard for, and security of, certain common freedoms. The functioning meaning of sexual freedoms given underneath is a commitment to the proceeding with discourse on common liberties connected with sexual wellbeing.

"The satisfaction of sexual wellbeing is attached to the degree to which basic liberties are regarded, secured and satisfied. Sexual freedoms embrace specific common liberties that are now perceived in worldwide and local basic liberties reports and other agreement archives and in public regulations.

Privileges basic to the acknowledgment of sexual wellbeing include:

the privileges to fairness and non-separation.

the option to be liberated from torment or to brutal, coldhearted or corrupting treatment or discipline.

the right to protection.

the freedoms to the most noteworthy feasible norm of wellbeing (counting sexual wellbeing) and government managed retirement.

the option to wed and to establish a family and go into marriage with the free and full assent of the planning mates, and to balance in and at the disintegration of marriage.

the option to choose the number and dividing of one's youngsters.

the freedoms to data, as well as instruction

the privileges to opportunity of assessment and articulation.

the right to a powerful solution for infringement of crucial freedoms.

The dependable work-out of common freedoms expects that all people regard the privileges of others.

The utilization of existing basic liberties to sexuality and sexual wellbeing comprise sexual freedoms. Sexual freedoms safeguard every one of individuals' privileges to satisfy and communicate their sexuality and appreciate sexual wellbeing, with due respect for the freedoms of others and inside a system of security against separation."

CHAPTER ONE

• SEXUAL WELLBEING

sexual wellbeing incorporates undeniably more than staying away from sickness or spontaneous pregnancy. We likewise accept that having a physically sent disease or undesirable pregnancy doesn't keep somebody from being or turning out to be physically sound.

Concocting a meaning of sexual wellbeing is a troublesome undertaking, as each culture, sub-culture, and individual has various principles of sexual wellbeing. Here's the meaning of sexual wellbeing:

Sexual wellbeing is the capacity to embrace and partake in our sexuality all through our lives. It is a significant piece of our physical and profound wellbeing. Being physically sound means:

Understanding that sexuality is a characteristic piece of life and includes more than sexual way of behaving.

Perceiving and regarding the sexual privileges we as a whole offer.

Approaching sexual wellbeing data, instruction, and care.

Trying to forestall accidental pregnancies and sexually transmitted diseases and look for care and treatment when required.

Having the option to encounter sexual delight, fulfillment, and closeness when wanted.

Having the option to discuss about sexual wellbeing with others including sexual accomplices and medical care suppliers.

• **SEXUAL WELLBEING ESSENTIALS**

Sexuality is important for being human. Love, friendship and closeness all assume a part in sound connections from youth through advanced age.

You frequently catch wind of the significance of physical, mental and profound wellbeing, however having positive expectations about your sexuality additionally is significant. Accomplishing sexual wellbeing considers:

Solid connections
Arranged pregnancies
Sickness anticipation

It's crucial for be very much educated pretty much all viewpoints regarding sexual wellbeing and the stuff to have a satisfying sexual coexistence. Also, it's critical to know about factors that can confuse your sexual wellbeing. Try not to allow humiliation to hold you back from raising worries or posing inquiries of your PCP or other medical services suppliers.

I.   SEXUALLY TRANSMITTED DISEASE COUNTERACTION

Physically communicated sicknesses (sexually transmitted diseases), or physically sent contaminations (STIs), are contaminations generally procured however unprotected sexual contact with somebody who's tainted.

In any case, you can't necessarily let know if somebody is tainted, in light of the fact that numerous STIs cause no side effects. Many individuals who have a STI don't have any acquaintance with it, truth be told.

That is the reason you must be cautious about STI avoidance. Boundary strategies for anti-conception medication, like condoms, additionally assist with lessening your gamble of getting most STIs. Assuming you're physically dynamic, having only one accomplice who consents to remain physically elite with you can likewise assist with forestalling STIs.

II. LADIES' SEXUAL WELLBEING

Sexual wellbeing is significant for a lady's prosperity, whether you're attempting to forestall pregnancy and physically sent diseases or you're stressed over low sex drive, difficult intercourse or different issues connected with ladies' sexual wellbeing.

Figure out how to accomplish a satisfying sexual relationship, and skill to safeguard yourself from physically communicated contaminations. As you age, grasp normal changes in ladies' sexual wellbeing — and how to keep a sound and pleasant sexual coexistence at whatever stage in life.

III. MEN'S SEXUAL WELLBEING

Sexual wellbeing is significant for a man's prosperity, whether you're attempting to forestall pregnancy and physically sent contaminations or you're stressed over erectile brokenness or different issues connected with men's sexual wellbeing.

For certain men, stresses over penis size top the rundown of their sexual wellbeing concerns. In any case, you're presumably surprisingly typical — and penis-development items and systems aren't probably going to be viable and may have chances.

As you age, figure out normal changes in men's sexual wellbeing — and how to keep a solid and pleasant sexual coexistence at whatever stage in life.

IV.   SEX AND MATURING

Grown-ups can remain physically dynamic no matter what their age. As a matter of fact, numerous more established grown-ups want and partake in a functioning sexual coexistence.

A continuous interest in sex, as well as fulfillment with the recurrence and nature of sexual movement, is decidedly connected with wellbeing in later life. Obviously, there are a few difficulties with regards to sex and maturing. Actual changes, sickness, handicaps and a few prescriptions can make sex testing or hard to appreciate.

There are numerous assets accessible to more seasoned grown-ups to assist them with accomplishing a wonderful sexual coexistence. Go ahead and raise worries with your PCP or other medical care supplier. Also, recollect, whatever your age, avoid potential risk to safeguard yourself from physically communicated contaminations.

V.   CONVERSING WITH KIDS ABOUT SEX

Children and sexuality — those words strike dread into the hearts of many guardians. However, conversing with kids about sex is a significant piece of nurturing. Youngsters and teenagers get a ton of data from companions and media sources, so they need your direction to assist them with settling on sound and fitting conclusions about their sexual way of behaving.

With regards to conversing with kids about sex, there's no standard content. Your choice to teach your kids about sexuality will probably be founded on the youngster's development, as well as your own objectives and values. Search for regular open doors and let your kid set the rhythm with their inquiries. As your kid develops, you can give more-definite reactions.

It's not unexpected to feel awkward while conversing with kids about sex. However, by giving exact and open correspondence, you increment the chances that your kid will comprehend your qualities and go with suitable decisions about sex.

CHAPTER TWO

• MANUAL FOR SEXUAL WELLBEING

At the point when somebody hears the expression, "sexual wellbeing," they might think it alludes just to staying away from a spontaneous pregnancy or forestalling Physically Sent Contaminations (STIs). While these areas are parts, sexual wellbeing is actually an umbrella term that incorporates numerous features of an individual's physical and close to home prosperity encompassing sex and sexuality.

WHAT ARE THE QUALITIES OF A PHYSICALLY SOUND INDIVIDUAL?

The American Sexual Wellbeing Affiliation characterizes somebody who is physically sound as having the

accompanying qualities, ways of behaving, and conviction frameworks around sex and connections:
They comprehend that sexuality is a characteristic piece of somebody's life and includes something other than sexual way of behaving.

Your sexuality is significantly more than your moxie (a.k.a sex drive). Some portion of understanding your sexuality is assuming command over your sexual wellbeing - this might incorporate, yet isn't restricted to, routinely getting tried for STIs and being on top of your regenerative wellbeing

They perceive that everybody has sexual freedoms.
Everybody has various inclinations — including who they like, what they appreciate physically, and how they decide to manage their body. It is critical to regard every individual's inclinations, regardless of whether they are not the same as your own!

They make protected, solid endeavors to forestall accidental pregnancy and STIs.

At the point when you decide to be physically dynamic, you additionally decide to assume on the liability of possibly becoming pregnant or potentially spreading or getting STIs. All things considered, dealing with your actual wellbeing (for example utilizing contraception and keeping up with great cleanliness) is essential for the security of both yourself and your accomplice.

They will use sexual wellbeing assets.

Being equipped with the fundamental data on the most proficient method to best take responsibility for sexual wellbeing will prompt you being an all the more physically solid individual generally. As a general rule, assets on points like assent, sexuality, and sex inspiration exist to assist people with turning out to be more sex positive.

They can encounter sexual joy, fulfillment, and closeness when they want.

Watchword here — "want." Somebody who is physically sound not just realizes that they are permitted to encounter sexual joy, yet in addition feels open to making limits (not having any desire to have intercourse is OK as well). Assent is provocative!

They can straightforwardly convey about their sexual wellbeing and requirements with private accomplices and medical services suppliers when required.

Being forthright about your sexual coexistence might appear to be startling, however it is essential to do as such to keep up with solid associations with yourself as well as other people. Furthermore, the more open you are with your medical services suppliers, the more probable you are to get the most ideal consideration.

These are commendable objectives to put and get together to focus on sexual wellbeing.

Not every person will actually want to scratch off every thing from the rundown, and that is not really a marker that they are deficient in sexual wellbeing or are generally undesirable.

In any case, by and large, security, both physical and profound, and satisfaction for everybody in a sexual relationship are the keys to living a physically sound, legitimate life. As a rule, sound people will communicate their own cravings while regarding the inclinations of others.

FOR WHAT REASON IS SEXUAL WELLBEING SO SIGNIFICANT?

Sexual wellbeing is significant in light of the fact that it empowers individuals people to assume responsibility for their regenerative wellbeing, and their close to home prosperity encompassing their personal connections. There are a few parts associated with turning out to be physically sound, some of which incorporate schooling, wellbeing, and correspondence (both with medical services suppliers and private accomplices)

Training

Sex training is shown in many schools all through the US. In any case, the educational plans normally shift and may just show understudies the chance of becoming pregnant or spreading STIs when they engage in sexual relations. So, people might have to assume control over sexual schooling to not just safeguard themselves from accidental pregnancy and STIs, yet additionally to gain proficiency with their own sexual inclinations.

Wellbeing

While examining sexual wellbeing, security is a term that might allude to counteraction of accidental pregnancy and STIs or insurance from sexual maltreatment. Physically solid people participate in safe sex rehearses.

While the most effective way to forestall impromptu preganancy is to rehearse forbearance (for example not engaging in sexual relations), this isn't practical for some indivdiuals. Fortunately, another fruitful strategy is carrying out contraception. Hormonal strategies, like the pill, fix, ring, and IUD, are extraordinary choices for ladies who need to have more prominent command over their conceptive wellbeing, as they are extremely viable at forestalling pregnancy when utilized as endorsed. In any case, these techniques don't shield people from the spread of STIs. Thusly, it is important to utilize an extra type of contraception, like condoms during penetrative sex (for example penis-to-vagina or penis-to-rear-end).

Tragically, there is no unequivocal method for forestalling sexual maltreatment, as this is extremely commonplace both in the US and all through the world. In any case, this doesn't imply that sex must be viewed as something frightening. Assuming you experience something that causes you to feel awkward, it is OK to stop. Sex ought to be agreeable for all interested parties and in the event that that isn't true, then something probably needs to change.

At the point when an individual turns out to be physically dynamic, they must speak with their PCPs and medical care group. While it might feel awkward to examine such a scary point, the more open you are, the more a medical services proficient will actually want to give educated, successful consideration. It is particularly vital to counsel a specialist in the event that you are thinking about hormonal contraception. When they have a thought of your wellbeing foundation and current way of life, they can endorse something they feel will be best for you.

Having solid correspondence with your partner is additionally significant. Connections flourish when the two accomplices are deferential, and impart their requirements, assumptions, and limits. A physically solid individual will feel happy with communicating genuineness to their accomplice whether this implies letting them know that they like or aversion a specific sex position, conceding to having a STI, or just expressing that you would rather not have intercourse. The more agreeable the two accomplices feel with one another, the more grounded a relationship can turn into.

CHAPTER THREE

• WHAT MAKES A SOLID SEXUAL RELATIONSHIP?

A sound sexual relationship spins around clear lines of correspondence more, the two accomplices ought to feel open to conveying what they like and aversion in regards to sex. As a rule, being in a sexual relationship ought to give you a feeling of prosperity, as it meets both your sexual and close to home necessities.

One more method for rehearsing great sexual wellbeing is by dealing with your body and doing taking part in exercises that cause you to feel erotic all alone. This might appear to be unique for each individual, yet a few strategies might incorporate cleaning up, buying a vibrator or other sex toys, and perusing or watching suggestive substance. It is absolutely sound and ordinary to embrace your longings. There is in many cases a negative disgrace around female mastubration, however it is an extraordinary device for investigating sexual joy, yet in addition for diminishing pressure.

Having a sound sexual relationship begins with dealing with yourself, When you find what encourages you, you can zero in on framing sound connections.

WHAT ARE THE RESULTS OF POOR SEXUAL WELLBEING?

Poor sexual wellbeing can prompt a large group of unfavorable outcomes. Absence of admittance to schooling or potentially assets can prompt accidental pregnancy and STIs.

Also, neglecting to speak with specialists can prompt long haul unexpected problems For example, it means a lot to open up to your medical services supplier about your sexual wellbeing, as they can assist you with ensuring it is in line. Essentially, captivating in a relationship that is unfulfilling can eventually cause poor psychological wellness and thus, decline one's general personal satisfaction. So, being straightforward both with your accomplice and yourself is a very vital piece of keeping up with great sexual wellbeing.

HOW MIGHT SOMEBODY WORK ON THEIR SEXUAL WELLBEING?

Some of the time, talking about delicate subjects to a sexual partner can be troublesome. Disgrace and negative social molding might make people overlook their requirements or those of their accomplice. At times, it could be helpful to address a specialist who is proficient and steady of sexual wellbeing.

A specialist can give an individual the devices they need to assist them with imparting their limits and assumptions consciously, and in a protected, sans judgment climate.

It's likewise essential to address a specialist about unambiguous sexual wellbeing needs. In the event that you are don't know where to begin, you can look at one of the numerous associations that exist to help people through their sexual wellbeing venture.

CHAPTER FOUR

• TIPS TO KEEP UP WITH YOUR SEXUAL WELLBEING

A solid sexual coexistence is very valuable for you!

It helps support insusceptibility, alleviates pressure and we should not fail to remember the positive state of mind endorphins. In any case, what's vital to comprehend is to know how to keep up with and further develop your sexual coexistence every day of the week. Take our relationship guidance and read on to be familiar with the main tips to keep up with your sexual wellbeing and have a solid sexual coexistence.

Perform Kegel practices for a superior sexual coexistence.

Kegel practices reinforce the PC muscles by expanding the progression of blood course in the pelvic locale, subsequently working on their tone and responsiveness. Solid PC muscles bring about more grounded sensations during excitement and climax. Pressing them during sex can improve the orgasmic delight for ladies.

This is the way to perform Kegel works out.

Most importantly, sit in a casual situation with your legs somewhat separated or rests on your back with the knees bowed and feet level on the floor. Presently concentration and begin getting the PC muscles as firmly as possible, 30 to 50 reiterations in quick progression. Inhale uninhibitedly all through. After this, agreement and hold the PC muscles for 5 seconds and afterward unwind for 5 seconds, slowly expanding this to 10 second compressions and 10 second unwinding. As you ace this, continue presenting varieties by holding the constrictions for longer terms with equivalent rest stretches.

Never treat sex as a weight.

The key falsehoods not in contemplating ways of denying it to your accomplice, yet to consider ways of being energetic about your sexual coexistence. It ought to be a functioning de-stressor in your life. All things considered, who couldn't cherish a decent sexual coexistence? Talk your accomplice into it assuming you are in the state of mind for it this evening.

 Allow things to like cleaning, making supper, going to work calls generally be gone to well in time. Flame light meals are old fashioned, we express dress down for it, wash up together and let the enthusiasm unfurl!

Express NO to smoking for a superior sexual coexistence.

 Nicotine in cigarettes is known to be the most compelling motivation for harming veins and conduits. Smoking prompts the harming of veins - indeed, even to the confidential pieces of the body. Restoratively talking, intense vasospasm, constriction of the penile tissue, and limited blood stream to the penis are repulsive impacts of smoking. As a matter of fact, cigarette smoking can likewise prompt male barrenness, by decreasing the nature of semen.

Make little motions with flawless timing.

Maturing feelings, mind and indifference toward sex can adversely influence an individual's sexual coexistence, whenever left uncontrolled and untreated. As age propels many individuals begin checking out their life. This might prompt disagreeable sentiments like existential tension, stress and wretchedness.

Hence, it is critical to do straightforward things with impeccable timing to uncover to her/him that you are as yet intrigued! Play with her while she is in the middle of cooking, or send him a sexual message from your telephone while he is caught up with completing a few somewhat late sends around evening time, cuddle with one another when you are staring at the TV together.

Try not to accept that the individual in question is the master.

As a rule, men like to flaunt that they are specialists at sex since they are frequently embarrassed to concede their frailty and naiveté. In this way, don't expect to be that he's the master. What's more, every one of the men out there, you should likewise not be held under the misleading deception of her being the master constantly. Discuss your longings with your accomplice and guarantee that it isn't generally the person in question driving.

Sex treatment can likewise attempt to keep up with your sexual wellbeing. Before you come to a choice to see a sex specialist, get some margin to dive in and investigate whether it is genuinely what you really want. Sex treatment won't show you how to have intercourse. All things being equal, it helps eliminate nerves, change mentalities and conduct, so typical reaction isn't repressed.

Presently you might ask what occurs in a sex treatment meeting.

Loads of individuals come to sex treatment after private conduct treatment fizzles, to assist them with their intersexual issues. Generally speaking sex treatment manages emotive issues, which hamper essential sexual issues. It additionally applies social proficiencies to manage the physiological side effects.

Remember to appreciate foreplay.

Despite the fact that you might be restless or energized, don't leap to it. Take as much time as necessary and give the other individual opportunity to heat up by enjoying broadened foreplay. Ensure you are plentifully excited before intercourse. Else sex can be even more a torment rather than delight and it can truly be a tragic encounter.

Deal with your maturing sexual coexistence really.

Your craving for sex might plunge as a result of the low degrees of testosterone in your body or in light old enough connected medical issue. Restoratively, it is recommended that you ought not be centered around accomplishing climax, yet you ought to begin partaking in one another's bodies and similarity.

Try not to depend a lot on superfluous medications and consistently make it a highlight converse with your PCP prior to beginning any new prescription daily practice, as it might have an unfriendly effect on your sexual craving. Jerking off, exotic back rubs, kissing, nestling and keeping up with open channels of correspondence are fundamental to resuscitate your advantage in sex.

Upgrade your sexual coexistence in the event that you are discouraged. A couple of ways of defeating wretchedness to upgrade sexual coexistence are:

- Work out your interests with the accomplice and attempt to consider commonly adequate and functional plans.

- Let yourself know that this is only a stage and your sexual coexistence will have returned to ordinary once you manage discouragement.

- Take mental treatment for discouragement.

- In the event that you don't wish to have total sex take a stab at enjoying exercises, for example, embracing, kissing and nestling as these may bring back the energy steadily.

- Try not to compress yourself into sex as this might exacerbate you.

- Assuming that you are on wretchedness meds, ask about the conceivable aftereffects on your sexual coexistence from your PCP.

Practice for that fiery sexual coexistence.

Practice is known for the majority medical advantages and one of them is most certainly sex. It helps fire up your blood dissemination by keeping your cardiovascular framework generous and cheerful. Wellbeing specialists all around the world accept that a lift in the degree of endorphins in the body helps love-production; also, being conditioned would clearly cause you and your accomplice to feel hotter prompting a more pleasurable encounter.

TOP 3 FOOD VARIETIES THAT WILL ASSIST WITH SUPPORTING YOUR SEXUAL COEXISTENCE:

Crude clams.

Distinguished as one of the highest level aphrodisiacs, crude clams help in setting the temperament. They are known for expanding the amount of sperm in men. That's what some say assuming you consolidate crude clams in your foreplay meeting, the tacky, disgusting kind of crude shellfish is sufficient to get you in that frame of mind.

Strawberries.

Enough has previously been said about how red aides in touching off energy. This red wet, drippy organic product makes for an amazing foreplay natural product. Dribble the juices over your accomplice's body and you'll in all actuality do fine and dandy.

Avocado.

Brimming with unsaturated fats, they are rich in folic corrosive which helps in using proteins in the body in this manner giving you more energy. They are to be sure amazing for your heart wellbeing and in the event that they are really great for your heart, they must be great for your sexual coexistence.

CHAPTER FIVE

• ANTI-CONCEPTION MEDICATION

CONTRACEPTION CHOICES: INTERESTING POINTS

Picking a technique for contraception can be troublesome. Know the choices and how to pick the kind of contraception that is appropriate for you.

In the event that you're thinking about utilizing conception prevention (contraception), you have different choices. To assist with picking the right technique for contraception for yourself as well as your accomplice, think about the accompanying inquiries.

What anti-conception medication choices are accessible?

Your contraception choices include:

Boundary techniques.

Models incorporate male and female condoms, as well as the stomach, cervical cap and prophylactic wipe.

Short-acting hormonal techniques.

Models incorporate anti-conception medication pills, as well as the vaginal ring (NuvaRing), skin fix (Xulane) and prophylactic infusion (Depo-Provera). These are viewed as short-acting techniques since you need to make sure to utilize them on a day to day, week after week or month to month premise.

Long-acting hormonal techniques.

Models incorporate the copper IUD (ParaGard), the hormonal IUD (Mirena, Skyla, Kyleena, others) and the prophylactic embed (Nexplanon). These are viewed as lengthy acting strategies since they keep going for three to 10 years after addition — contingent upon the gadget — or until you choose to have the gadget eliminated.

Sanitization.

This is a super durable technique for conception prevention. Models incorporate tubal ligation for ladies and vasectomy for men.

Spermicide or vaginal gel.

These are nonhormonal choices for anti-conception medication. Spermicide is a sort of prophylactic that kills sperm or prevents it from moving. Vaginal pH controller gel (Phexxi) prevents sperm from moving, so they can't get to an egg to treat it. You put these items in the vagina just before sex.

Ripeness mindfulness techniques.

These strategies center around knowing which days of the month you can get pregnant (fruitful), frequently founded on basal internal heat level and cervical bodily fluid. To try not to get pregnant, you don't engage in sexual relations nearby the days you are prolific, or you utilize a boundary strategy for conception prevention.

It's additionally essential to know about crisis contraception — like a next day contraceptive (Plan B One-Step, Aftera, ella, others) — which can be utilized to forestall pregnancy after unprotected sex.

How do the different contraception choices function? Different kinds of contraception work in various ways. Contraception techniques may:

Keep sperm from arriving at the egg

Inactivate or harm sperm

Keep an egg from being delivered every month

Modify the covering of the uterus so a treated egg doesn't join to it

Thicken cervical bodily fluid so sperm can only with significant effort go through it

What is the strategy's viability?

To be successful, some technique for contraception should be utilized reliably and accurately. Contraceptives that require little exertion from you, like IUDs, preventative inserts and disinfection, are related with lower pregnancy rates. Interestingly, strategies that require checking ripeness or occasional restraint are related with higher pregnancy rates.

Is it reversible?

The technique for contraception you pick relies upon your regenerative objectives. In the event that you're arranging pregnancy sooner rather than later, you might need a strategy that is effectively halted or rapidly reversible, like a short-acting hormonal technique or an obstruction technique. To forestall pregnancy for a more drawn out measure of time, you might think about a long-acting strategy, like an IUD. If you're sure that you would rather not get pregnant whenever later on, you might lean toward a long-lasting technique, like disinfection. You might find that different preventative choices work for you at various phases of your life.

Is it viable with your strict convictions or social practices?

A few types of contraception are viewed as an infringement of specific strict regulations or social practices. Gauge the dangers and advantages of a conception prevention technique against your own convictions.

Is it helpful and reasonable?

It's essential to pick a sort of contraception that suits your way of life. For certain individuals, the most helpful type of anti-conception medication might be one that is not difficult to utilize, makes no irksome side impacts or doesn't upset the sexual experience. For other people, accommodation implies no solution is required. While picking a strategy for conception prevention, consider that you are so able to prepare or follow an inflexible prescription timetable.

A few techniques for contraception are reasonable, while others are more expensive. Get some information about your inclusion, and afterward consider the cost as you settle on a choice.

What are the aftereffects?

Consider your capacity to bear the conceivable incidental effects related with a specific contraception strategy. A few techniques present more incidental effects — some possibly serious — than others. Converse with your PCP about your clinical history and what it could mean for your decision of anti-conception medication.

Does it safeguard against physically sent diseases?

Male and female condoms are the main strategies for anti-conception medication that offer solid insurance from physically sent diseases. Except if you are in a commonly monogamous relationship and have been tried for physically sent contaminations, utilize another condom each time you have intercourse notwithstanding some other strategy for contraception you use.

Does it offer different advantages?

As well as forestalling pregnancy, a few contraceptives give advantages like more unsurprising, lighter feminine cycles, a diminished gamble of physically sent diseases or a decrease in the gamble of certain malignant growths. Assuming that these advantages are critical to you, they might impact your decision of conception prevention choice.

Is it adequate to your sexual accomplice?

Your accomplice might have contraception inclinations that are like or unique in relation to your own. Talk about contraception choices with your accomplice to assist with figuring out which technique is OK to both of you.

How would I pick?

The best technique for anti-conception medication for you is one that is protected, that you are open to utilizing, and that you can utilize reliably and accurately. Your favored technique for anti-conception medication might change over your lifetime and is impacted by various variables, including:

Your age and wellbeing history

Your conceptive objectives, for example, the quantity of kids you need and how soon you need to get pregnant

Relationship factors, including conjugal status, number of sexual accomplices, how frequently you have intercourse and accomplice inclinations

Strict convictions

Contrasts between contraception strategies, including how compelling they are at forestalling pregnancy, aftereffects, cost and whether they forestall physically communicated diseases

Realizing your choices is certainly essential for the choice cycle — however a genuine evaluation of yourself and your connections is similarly as significant while concluding which kind of contraception is appropriate for you.

CHAPTER SIX

• CONCLUSION

Assuming you're hoping to keep up with sexual action in bed the entire evening, you're in good company.

Numerous men are searching for ways of improving their sexual execution. This can incorporate working on existing issues or looking for better approaches to keep your accomplice cheerful.

There are a lot of male improvement pills available, however there are numerous straightforward ways of remaining firmer and last longer without visiting the drug store.

Remember that your penis deals with pulse, and ensure your circulatory framework is working at top shape.

Fundamentally, what's great for your heart is really great for your sexual wellbeing.

Continue to peruse to track down other simple methods for working on your sexual execution.

1. Remain dynamic

One of the most outstanding ways of further developing your wellbeing is cardiovascular activity. Sex could get your pulse up, yet standard activity can help your sexual presentation by keeping your heart in shape.

Thirty minutes per day of sweat-breaking exercise, like running and swimming, can do miracles to help your moxie.

2. Eat these foods grown from the ground

Certain food varieties can likewise assist you with expanding blood stream. They include:

Onions and garlic.

These food sources may not be perfect for your breath, but rather they can help your blood flow.

Bananas.

This potassium-rich natural product can assist with bringing down your circulatory strain, which can help your significant sexual parts and lift sexual execution.

Chilies and peppers.

All-regular zesty food sources assist your blood with streaming by lessening hypertension and aggravation.

3. Eat these meats and different food varieties

Here are a few additional food varieties that can assist you with accomplishing better blood stream:

Omega-3 unsaturated fats.

This kind of fat increments blood stream. You can think that it is in salmon, fish, avocados, and olive oil.

Vitamin B-1. T

his nutrient assists signals in your sensory system with moving faster, including signals from your cerebrum to your penis. It's tracked down in pork, peanuts, and kidney beans.

Eggs.

High in other B nutrients, eggs assist with adjusting chemical levels. This can diminish pressure that frequently restrains an erection.

4. Diminish pressure

Stress can influence all region of your wellbeing, including your charisma.

Stress expands your pulse (in the awful way) and increments circulatory strain. Both of these are harming to sexual longing and execution.

Mental pressure can likewise influence accomplishing an erection or arriving at a climax.

Practice is an incredible method for decreasing pressure and work on your wellbeing.

Conversing with your accomplice about your pressure can likewise quiet you down, while reinforcing your relationship simultaneously.

Stress can likewise set off persistent vices, for example, smoking or liquor utilization, which can hurt your sexual execution.

5. Overcome terrible vices

What you depend on to loosen up, like smoking and drinking liquor, could likewise influence sexual execution.

While studies recommend that a little red wine can further develop flow, an excess of liquor can make unfavorable impacts.

Energizers thin veins and have been connected to feebleness. Chopping down or stopping smoking is perhaps the earliest move toward further develop execution.

Supplanting negative behavior patterns with sound ones, like activity and eating great, can assist with helping sexual wellbeing.

6. Get some sun

Daylight stops the body's creation of melatonin. This chemical assists us with resting yet additionally calms our sexual desires. Less melatonin implies the potential for more sexual longing.

Getting outside and allowing the sun to hit your skin can assist with awakening your sex drive, particularly throughout the cold weather months when the body creates more melatonin.

7. Jerk off to further develop life span

On the off chance that you're not enduring insofar as you'd like in bed, you could require some training. While sex is the most ideal way to rehearse for sex, masturbation can likewise assist you with working on your life span.

In any case, how you stroke off could make unfavorable impacts. Assuming that you hurry through it, you could coincidentally diminish the time you last with your accomplice. The mystery is making it last, very much like you need to when you're in good company.

8. Focus on your accomplice

Sex is definitely not a road that goes only one direction. Really focusing on your accomplice's longings makes sex pleasurable for them, yet it can likewise assist with turning you on or dial you back. Discussing this in advance can assist with facilitating any clumsiness on the off chance that you want to dial back during a warmed second.

Substituting speed or zeroing in on your accomplice while you have some time off can make for a more charming encounter for both of you.

9. Get more assistance assuming you really want it
Assuming you have erectile brokenness, Peyronie's infection, or other analyzed messes, you might require clinical treatment. Make sure to your primary care physician about how you can work on your sexual execution.

It's never a terrible choice to work out, eat right, and partake in your sexual coexistence without limit.

www.ingramcontent.com/pod-product-compliance
Lightning Source LLC
Chambersburg PA
CBHW060212260726
48658CB00005BA/2006